Homemade Soap Making

Soap Making Book with Simple and Gentle Soap Recipes for Sensitive Skin

Homemade Soaps

Book 2

Janela Maccsone

Text Copyright © [Janela Maccsone]

All rights reserved. No part of this guide may be reproduced in any form without permission in writing from the publisher except in the case of brief quotations embodied in critical articles or reviews.

Legal & Disclaimer

The information contained in this book and its contents is not designed to replace or take the place of any form of medical or professional advice; and is not meant to replace the need for independent medical, financial, legal or other professional advice or services, as may be required. The content and information in this book has been provided for educational and entertainment purposes only.

The content and information contained in this book has been compiled from sources deemed reliable, and it is accurate to the best of the Author's knowledge, information, and belief. However, the Author cannot guarantee its accuracy and validity and cannot be held liable for any errors and/or omissions. Further, changes are periodically made to this book as and when needed. Where appropriate and/or necessary, you must consult a professional (including but not limited to your doctor, attorney, financial advisor or such other professional advisor) before using any of the suggested remedies, techniques, or information in this book.

Upon using the contents and information contained in this book, you agree to hold harmless the Author from and against any damages, costs, and expenses, including any legal fees potentially resulting from the application of any of the information provided by this book. This disclaimer applies to any loss, damages or injury caused by the use and application, whether directly or indirectly, of any advice or information presented, whether for breach of contract, tort, negligence, personal injury, criminal intent, or under any other cause of action.

You agree to accept all risks of using the information presented in this book.

You agree that by continuing to read this book, where appropriate and/or necessary, you shall consult a professional (including but not limited to your doctor, attorney, or financial advisor or such other advisor as needed) before using any of the suggested remedies, techniques, or information in this book.

ISBN: 9798588125161

Homemade Soaps 5

Kitchen Tools 6

Tips and Tricks 7

Chapter 1: Hot Process Soaps 8

Homemade Lemon Soap 8

Sensitive Skin Almond Soap 10

Honey and Orange Soap 12

Handmade Raspberry-Coconut Soap 14

Handmade Orange and Cherry Soap 16

Delicate Blueberry Soap 18

Mild Cinnamon Soap 20

Homemade Green Tea and Lavender Soap 22

Handmade Strawberry-Coconut Soap 24

Coconut Soap for Sensitive Skin 26

Homemade Peach Soap 27

Mild Almond Milk Soap 29

Chapter 2: Cold Process Soaps 31

Rose Soap 31

Cinnamon and Pineapple Soap 33

Handmade Mango and Coconut Soap 34

Orange and Honey Soap 35

Mild Coconut Soap 37

Peach and Almond Soap 38

Handmade Orange and Patchouli Soap 39

Homemade Pineapple Soap 40

Pears-Almond Soap 42

Handmade Goat's Milk and Coconut Soap 43

Banana and Honey Soap 45

Rose-Coconut Soap 47

Apple and Honey Soap 49

Milk Soap 51

Cherry and Coconut Soap 53

Activated Charcoal Soap 54

Gooseberry Soap 56

Mild Carrot Soap 57

Handmade Coffee Soap 59

Lemon Soap for Dry Skin 60

Grapefruit Soap for Clean Skin 62

Orange and Grapefruit Soap with Honey 64

Apricot Soap with Lemon 66

Blueberry Soap 68

Yogurt and Avocado Soap 70

Raspberry Soap 72

Cheery and Grapefruit Soap 73

Conclusion 75

Homemade Soaps

The popularity of handmade soap is growing every day due to the exclusivity and naturalness.

Handmade soap is always an exclusive, handmade product. Making homemade soap is a fun, creative and completely uncomplicated process!

You don't need to be a professional soap maker to use soap recipes from this book and to prepare soap for yourself, your friends and family. We would like to encourage you to test various soap recipes and to experiment adding your own colors and flavors!

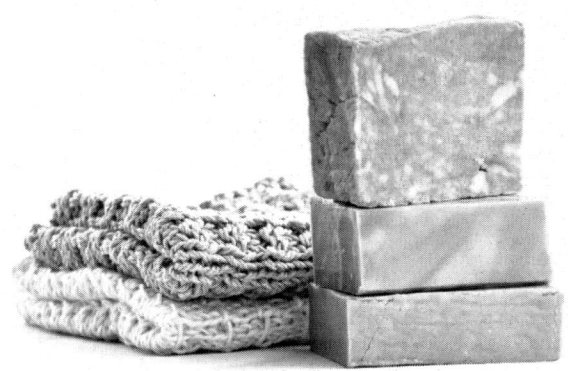

Kitchen Tools

To prepare high-quality homemade soaps you will need to have the right kitchen utensils. The following list of kitchen instruments will help you to organize your soap making process.

- a bowl (plastic, heat resistant or stainless steel) that can withstand high temperatures;
- few pots;
- stick blender or food processor;
- potato masher or fork;
- burner or kitchen stove;
- sharp knife to cut the soap into pieces;
- zip-lock bags;
- soap molds;

Tips and Tricks

- Before starting the soap preparation process, visualise and think about the soap you would like to have. It is better to have a clear plan;
- Mix essential oils in the separate containers, bowls or pots;
- Do not hurry and get the soap out of the molds carefully.

Chapter 1: Hot Process Soaps

Homemade Lemon Soap

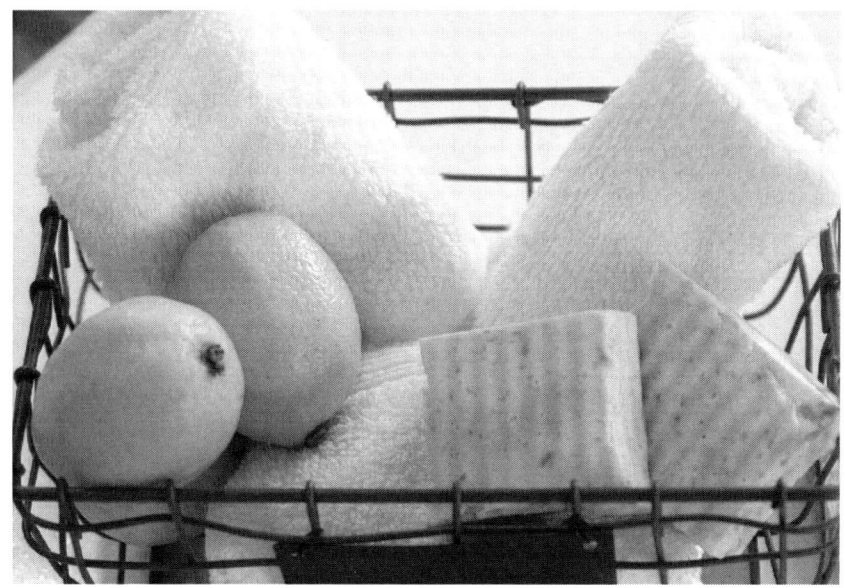

Prep Time: about 70-80 minutes

Cooking Time: 65 minutes

Ingredients:

- 5 dried lemon slices
- 1 tablespoon lemon zest, minced
- 22 oz coconut oil
- 11 oz olive oil
- 0.8 cup of palm oil
- 1 tablespoon vitamin A
- 1.5 cup of water
- 6 oz lye

How to Make Homemade Soap:

1. Spoon the lemon zest into the warm water and mix.

2. Carefully spoon the lye into the water with the lemon zest and mix well. The fumes will be produced during the lye melting process. Wear the rubber gloves, goggles and breathing mask.

3. Let the lye to cool for around half an hour. Place the lye into the well-ventilated room or on the balcony.

4. Pour the coconut oil into the pot. Then pour the olive oil and palm oil and stir well. Melt the oils over the low heat for around 20 minutes. Keep stirring well to prevent oils from burning.

5. Then slowly pour the lye and water mixture into the oils and mix well.

6. Boil the lye and oils mixture over the low heat for about 45 minutes. Keep stirring to prevent the soap batter from burning and rising. After 45 minutes of boiling set the lemon soap batter aside to cool it.

7. Use a PH test to check if the soap is ready. Ideal values are between 7 and 10. If the indicator is higher than 10, then this means that the soap is not ready.

8. Pour the vitamin A. Combine all the ingredients and blend using a stick blender. Blend the lemon soap batter until there is a smooth consistency and homogenous mass.

9. Place the dried lemon slices on the bottom of the molds. Then pour the soap batter into the few molds. In 20-24 hours take the soap out of the molds and cut it into pieces. You can use the soap after two or three weeks.

Remember! During the soap preparation process always use rubber gloves, goggles, long sleeves and breathing mask.

Sensitive Skin Almond Soap

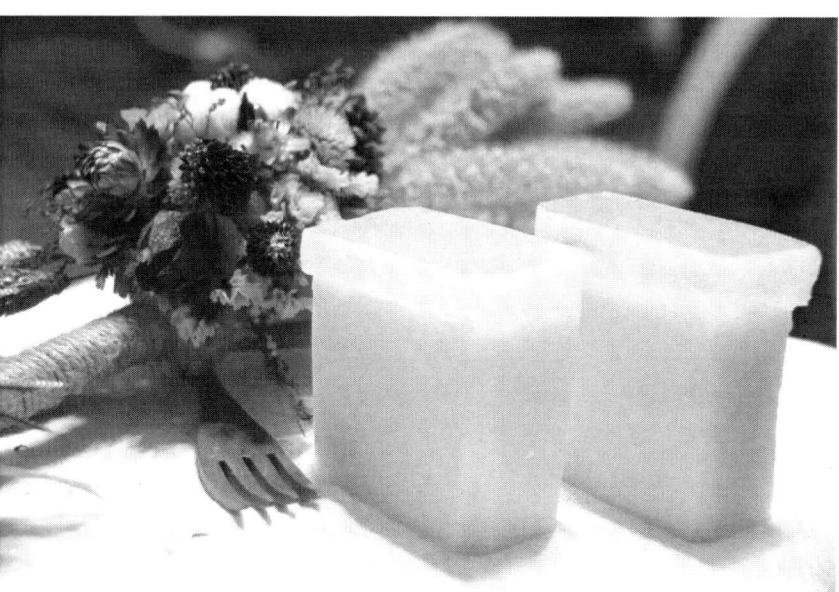

Prep Time: approximately 50 minutes

Boiling Time: 20 minutes

Ingredients:

- 4 tablespoons almond oil
- 21 oz coconut oil
- 12 oz olive oil
- 6 oz castor oil
- 1 tablespoon vitamin E
- 10 oz water
- 5 oz lye

How to Make Homemade Soap:

1. Slowly pour the lye into the water and mix well until there is a smooth consistency. Let it cool for around 20-30 minutes. Place the mixture into the well-ventilated room or on the balcony.
2. In a pot, mix the coconut oil with the olive oil and castor oil. Boil the oils on the burner for around 15 minutes.
3. Pour the lye and water mixture into the oils and mix well.

4. Boil the lye and oils mixture over the low heat for about 40 minutes. Then set the soap batter aside to cool it.

5. Use a PH test to check if the soap is ready. The values should stay between 7 and 10.

6. Then pour the sweet almond oil and vitamin E and blend well until there is a smooth consistency and homogenous mass.

7. Pour the soap batter into the molds. In 24 hours you can take your soap out of the molds and cut it into the bars. Wait for two or three weeks until the process of the saponification will complete and only then use your almond soap.

Remember! During the soap preparation process always use rubber gloves, goggles, long sleeves and breathing mask.

Honey and Orange Soap

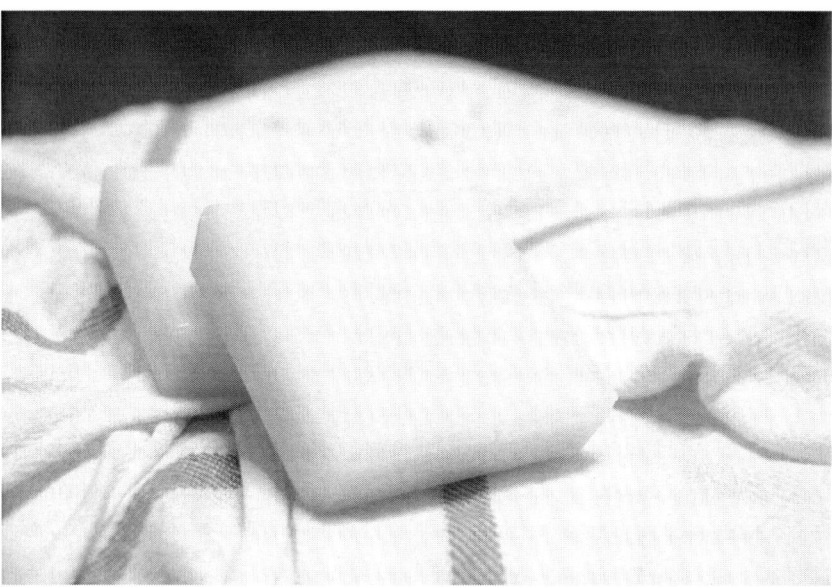

Prep Time: about 60-70 minutes

Cooking Time: 50 minutes

Ingredients:

- 5 oz orange fragrance oil
- 4 oz honey
- 22 oz coconut oil
- 17 oz olive oil
- 5 oz palm oil
- 10 oz distilled water
- 5.5 oz lye

How to Make Homemade Soap:

1. First, slowly spoon the lye into the water and mix well until there is a smooth consistency. Remember that the fumes will be produced during this process, so don't forget to wear the rubber gloves, goggles and breathing mask. Let it cool for around 20 minutes.

2. In a pot, combine the oils. Melt the oils on a burner 20 minutes and keep stirring.

3. Pour the lye and water mixture into the oils and stir well.

4. Cook the lye and oils mixture over the low heat for about 30 minutes. Keep stirring to prevent the soap batter from burning and rising. Cool the batter.

5. Check if the soap is ready using a PH test. Ideal values are between 7 and 10.

6. Spoon the honey and orange oil. Mix all the ingredients using a stick blender until there is a homogenous mass.

7. Pour the orange soap batter into the molds. In 24 hours take the soap out of the molds and cut it into pieces. Wait for two or three weeks and use the soap.

Handmade Raspberry-Coconut Soap

Prep Time: approximately 80-90 minutes

Boiling Time: 75 minutes

Ingredients:

- 1 cup of fresh raspberries
- 21 oz coconut oil
- 15 oz olive oil
- 5 oz castor oil
- 2 tablespoons shredded coconut
- 10 oz water
- 5.5 oz lye

How to Make Homemade Soap:

1. In a pot, cook the raspberries over low heat for 20 minutes and skim the foam. Then mash the raspberries using the potato masher and cool for half an hour in the well-ventilated place.

2. Slowly pour the lye into the water and mix well. Let it cool for around 20-30 minutes.

3. In a pot, mix the coconut oil with the olive oil and castor oil. Boil the oils on the burner for around 15 minutes.

4. Pour the lye and water mixture into the oils and mix well.

5. Boil the lye and oils mixture with the raspberries over medium heat for about 40 minutes and keep stirring to prevent the soap batter from burning.

6. Use a PH test to check if the soap is ready. The values between 7 and 10.

7. Mix in the shredded coconut and blend using a stick blender.

8. Pour the soap batter into the molds. In 24 hours take your soap out of the molds and cut it into the square pieces. Wait for two or three weeks until the process of the saponification will complete and only then use the soap.

Remember! During the soap preparation process always use rubber gloves, goggles, long sleeves and breathing mask.

Handmade Orange and Cherry Soap

Prep Time: about 1 hour

Melting Time: 20 minutes

Ingredients:

- 1 tablespoon orange zest, minced
- 2 tablespoons orange essential oil
- 15 oz cherry kernel oil
- 12 oz coconut oil
- 10 oz olive oil
- 5 oz palm oil
- 1.5 cup of water
- 6 oz lye

How to Make Homemade Soap:

1. Spoon the orange zest into the warm water and mix well to.
2. Carefully spoon the lye into the water with the orange zest and mix well.
3. The fumes will be produced during the lye melting process. Wear the rubber gloves, goggles and breathing mask.
4. Let the lye to cool for around one hour. Place the lye into the well-ventilated room or on the balcony.
5. In a pot, combine the coconut, olive and palm oils and stir well. Melt the oils over the low heat for around 30 minutes. Keep stirring well to prevent them from burning.
6. Then slowly pour the lye and water mixture into the oils and mix well.
7. Boil the lye and oils mixture over the low heat for about 45 minutes. Keep stirring to prevent the soap batter from burning and rising. Then cool the soap batter.
8. Use a PH test to check if the soap is ready. Ideal values are between 7 and 10. If the indicator is higher than 10, then this means that the soap is not ready.
9. Add the cherry kernel oil and orange essential oil. Blend using a stick blender until there is a smooth consistency and pureed mass.

10. Pour the soap batter into the molds. In 20-24 hours take the soap out of the molds and cut it into pieces. You can use the soap after two or three weeks. Give the soap some time to "rest".

Remember! During the soap preparation process always use rubber gloves, goggles, long sleeves and breathing mask.

Delicate Blueberry Soap

Prep Time: approximately 65-70 minutes

Cooking Time: 60-65 minutes

Ingredients:

- 1 cup of fresh blueberries
- 19 oz olive oil
- 16 oz palm oil
- 11 oz castor oil
- 8 oz shea butter
- 2 drops blue soap colorant
- 12 oz water
- 6 oz lye

How to Make Homemade Soap:

1. In a bowl, mash the blueberries using a potato masher. Then transfer the blueberries to a pot and boil over low heat for 20 minutes. Skim the foam. Keep stirring to prevent blueberries from burning.

2. Carefully spoon the lye into the water and mix well until there is a smooth consistency and homogenous mass. Remember that the fumes will be produced during this process, so don't forget to wear the rubber gloves. Cool the lye for around half an hour.

3. Meanwhile, in a pot, combine the oils. Pour the olive oil, palm oil and castor oil and mix well. Then spoon the shea butter and melt the oils and butter over the low heat for 15-20 minutes.

4. Put on a mask, rubber gloves and goggles and slowly pour the lye and water mixture into the oils and mix well.

5. Mix in the blue soap colorant into the lye and oils mixture and blend using a stick blender until there is a creamy and pureed consistency.

6. Melt the lye and oils mixture over the medium heat for about 25 minutes. Keep stirring to prevent the soap batter from burning and rising.

7. Use a PH test to check if the soap is ready. Ideal values are between 7 and 10. If higher than 10, then cook for 10 minutes and check once more time.

8. Slowly pour the blueberries and puree the ingredients.

9. Pour the blueberry soap batter into the silicon molds. After one or two days take your soap out of the molds. Leave the soap in the well-ventilated room for 10 days and then use it. The soap needs some time because the saponification process should end.

Always remember, that during the soap preparation process wear rubber gloves, goggles, long sleeves and breathing mask.

Mild Cinnamon Soap

Prep Time: approximately 2 hours

Cooking Time: 55 minutes

Ingredients:

- 7 drops cinnamon essential oil
- 17 oz olive oil
- 11 oz palm oil
- 6 oz castor oil
- 4 oz cocoa butter
- 11 oz distilled water
- 6 oz lye

How to Make Homemade Soap:

1. First, carefully spoon the lye into the water and mix well until there is a smooth consistency. Remember that the fumes will be produced during this process, so wear the rubber gloves, goggles and breathing mask. Cool for around 30 minutes.
2. In a pot, combine the oils: olive oil, palm oil and castor oil. Melt the oils on a burner for around 20 minutes. Spoon the cocoa butter and stir well.
3. Pour the lye and water mixture into the oils and blend using a stick blender until there is a homogenous and pureed consistency.
4. Boil over the low heat for about 40 minutes. Keep stirring to prevent the soap batter from burning and rising. Then cool the soap batter.
5. Use a PH test to check if the soap is ready. Ideal values are between 7 and 10. If the indicator is higher than 10, then cook further.
6. Pour the cinnamon essential oil. Mix the oils and lye well. You can use a stick blender or a food processor.
7. Pour the cinnamon soap batter into the molds. In 24 hours take your soap out of the molds and cut it into the square pieces. Then wait for 8-10 days and start using the cinnamon soap.

Always remember! During the soap preparation process use rubber gloves, goggles, long sleeves and breathing mask. It is a must.

Homemade Green Tea and Lavender Soap

Prep Time: approximately 60-65 minutes

Cooking Time: 50 minutes

Ingredients:

- 2 tablespoons green tea leaves, ground
- 10 drops Green tea oil
- 10 oz lavender essential oil
- 16 oz olive oil
- 11 oz palm oil
- 6 oz castor oil
- 5 oz raw cocoa butter
- 11 oz distilled water
- 6 oz 100% pure lye

How to Make Homemade Soap:

1. Pour the lye into the water and mix well until there is a smooth consistency and homogenous mass. Remember that the fumes will be produced during this process. Then cool for around half an hour.

2. In a pot, combine the olive oil, palm oil and castor oil. Melt the oils on a burner for around 10 minutes. Keep stirring to prevent oils from burning. Spoon the cocoa butter and melt with the oils for 10 minutes until the butter dissolves completely. Stir well until you get a homogeneous mass and creamy consistency.

3. Pour the lye and water mixture into the oils and cocoa butter mixture and mix well. Add the tea leaves.

4. Boil the lye, tea leaves and oils mixture over the low heat for about 30 minutes and then set the soap batter to cool.

5. Use a PH test to check if the soap is ready. Ideal values are between 7 and 10.

6. Pour the Green tea oil and lavender essential oil. Beat the ingredients with a blender until there is a smooth consistency and homogenous mass.

7. Pour the soap batter into the molds. In 24 hours take the green tea and lavender soap out of the molds and cut it into the square pieces. Then wait two or three weeks and start using your soap.

Remember! During the soap preparation process always use rubber gloves, goggles, long sleeves and breathing mask.

Handmade Strawberry-Coconut Soap

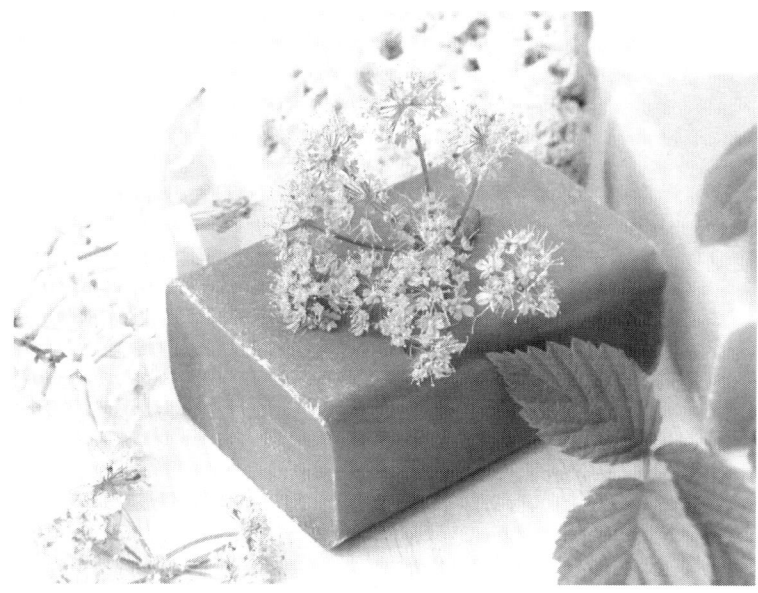

Prep Time: about 70-80 minutes

Boiling Time: 60 minutes

Ingredients:

- 3 tablespoons strawberry essential oil
- 15 oz coconut oil
- 12 oz olive oil
- 6 oz palm oil
- 2 tablespoons shredded coconut
- 10 oz water
- 5.5 oz lye

How to Make Homemade Soap:

1. Slowly pour the lye into the water and mix well. Let it cool for around half an hour.
2. In a pot, mix the coconut oil with the olive oil and palm oil. Boil the oils over the low heat for 15-20 minutes.
3. Pour the lye and water mixture into the oils and mix well.

4. Boil the lye and oils over medium heat for about 40 minutes. Keep stirring to prevent the soap batter from burning.
5. Use a PH test to check if the soap is ready. The values should be between 7 and 10.
6. Add in the shredded coconut and strawberry essential oil. Then blend the soap batter using a stick blender.
7. Pour the soap batter into the few molds. In 24 hours take your soap out of the molds and cut it into the pieces. Wait for two or three weeks until the process of the saponification will complete and only then use the soap.

During the soap preparation process always use rubber gloves, goggles, long sleeves and breathing mask.

Coconut Soap for Sensitive Skin

Prep Time: about 50 minutes

Boiling Time: 20 minutes

Ingredients:

- 22 oz coconut oil
- 13 oz palm oil
- 7 oz castor oil
- 5 oz coconut butter
- 10 oz water
- 5 oz lye

How to Make Homemade Soap:

1. Slowly pour the lye into the water. Stir until smooth. Cool for around half an hour. Place the mixture into the well-ventilated room or on the balcony.

2. In a pot, mix the coconut oil with the palm oil and castor oil. Boil the oils on the burner for around 20 minutes and spoon the coconut butter. Cook for 10 minutes or longer until the coconut butter melts. Stir all the time.

3. Pour the lye and water mixture into the oils and mix well.

4. Boil the lye and oils mixture over the low heat for about 40 minutes.

5. Cool the batter and check if the soap is ready by using a PH test. The values should stay between 7 and 10.

6. After positive PH test pour the soap batter into the molds. In 24 hours take the soap out of the molds and cut it into the bars. Wait for two or three weeks until the process of the saponification will complete and only then use the coconut soap.

Remember! During the soap preparation process always use rubber gloves, goggles, long sleeves and breathing mask.

Homemade Peach Soap

Prep Time: about 85 minutes

Cooking Time: 70-75 minutes

Ingredients:

- 3 peaches, pitted and diced
- 8 drops peach fragrance oil
- 1 teaspoon orange soap colorant
- 18 oz olive oil
- 16 oz palm oil
- 13 oz castor oil
- 10 oz shea butter
- 10 oz distilled water
- 7 oz 100% pure lye

How to Make Homemade Soap:

1. Put on a mask, rubber gloves and goggles and carefully spoon the lye into the water and mix well until there is a smooth consistency and homogenous mass. Cool the lye and water mixture for 20 minutes in the cold and ventilated place.

2. Then, in a pot, combine the olive, palm and castor oils. Melt the oils over the medium heat for 10 minutes. Spoon the shea butter and melt for 10 minutes until the butter dissolves completely. Keep stirring all the time to prevent the oils from burning.

3. Meanwhile, cook the peaches with some water over the low heat for about 20 minutes. Keep stirring to prevent the peaches from burning. Skim the foam while boiling.

4. Then blend the peaches with a blender until pureed consistency.

5. Slowly pour the lye and water mixture into the oils and stir well.

6. Combine the orange soap colorant and pureed peaches with the lye and oils mixture and blend using a stick blender until there is a creamy consistency and homogenous mass.

7. Cook the lye and oils mixture over the low heat for about 30 minutes. Keep stirring to prevent the soap batter from burning and rising.

8. Use a PH test to check if the soap is ready.

9. Then mix in the peach fragrance oil and blend the ingredients well.

10. Ladle the peach soap into the silicon molds. In 22-24 hours take the peach soap out of the molds and cut it into the medium bars. Leave the soap in the well-ventilated room or on the balcony for few weeks. After two or three weeks you are free to start using the fragrant peach soap. Give the soap some time to "rest".

Remember! During the soap preparation process always use rubber gloves, goggles, long sleeves and breathing mask.

Mild Almond Milk Soap

Prep Time: about 1 hour

Melting Time: 20 minutes

Ingredients:

- 10 drops almond oil
- 20 oz coconut oil
- 11 oz olive oil
- 7 oz of palm oil
- 2 tablespoons shea butter
- 1 tablespoon vitamin E
- 1.5 cup of almond milk
- 6 oz lye

How to Make Homemade Soap:

1. Pour the almond milk into the stainless steel bowl and place it into the sink with ice and cold water. Then slowly add the lye into the almond milk and mix well. The fumes will be produced during the lye melting process, so wear the rubber gloves, goggles and breathing mask.
2. Let the lye to cool for around half an hour. Leave the lye in the cold and ventilated room or on the balcony.
3. In the pot, combine the coconut oil with the olive oil, palm oil and shea butter. Melt the soap ingredients over the low heat for around 20 minutes. Keep stirring well to prevent oils and shea butter from burning.
4. Then slowly pour the lye and almond milk mixture into the oils and mix well.
5. Boil the lye and oils mixture over the low heat for about 15-20 minutes. Keep stirring to prevent the soap batter from burning and rising.
6. Use a PH test to check if the soap is ready. Ideal values are between 7 and 10.

7. Spoon the vitamin E and add the almond oil. Whisk until smooth and creamy.

8. Then pour the soap batter into the round molds. In 22-24 hours take the soap out of the molds and cut it into pieces. You can use the soap after two or three weeks when the saponification process is over.

Remember! During the soap preparation process always use rubber gloves, goggles, long sleeves and breathing mask.

Chapter 2: Cold Process Soaps

Rose Soap

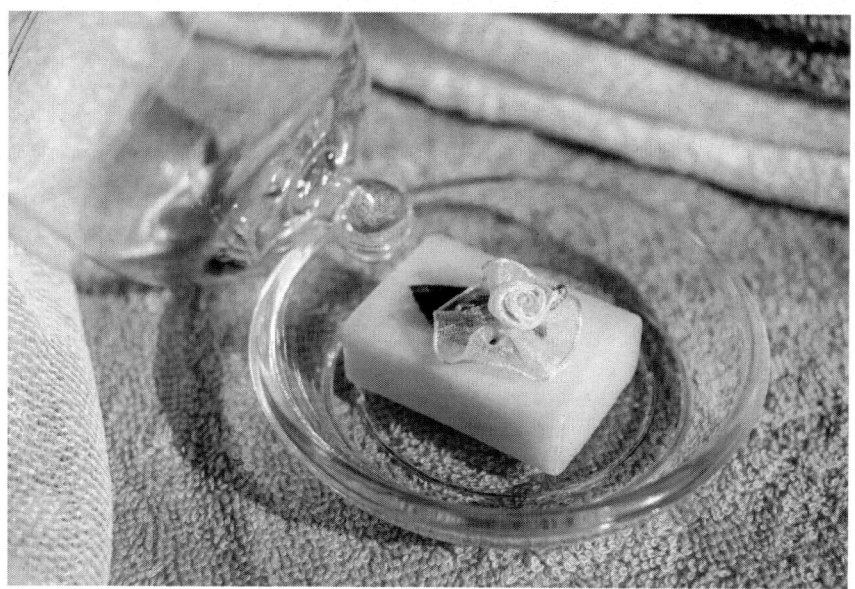

Prep Time: 50-60 minutes

Ingredients:

- 20 drops rose essential oil
- 4 drops pink soap colorant
- 23 oz palm oil
- 22 oz canola oil
- 5 oz shea butter
- 7 oz 100% pure lye
- 15 oz distilled water

How to Make Homemade Soap:

1. Slowly spoon the lye into the water and mix well until the lye dissolves. Wear the rubber gloves, goggles and breathing mask, because the fumes will be produced.

2. Cool the lye and water for around half an hour until the inner temperature of the mixture reaches 95 degrees Fahrenheit. Leave the mixture in the ventilated place and forget about it for 30 minutes or even longer.

3. Meanwhile, combine the palm oil and canola oil and melt them over the low heat for around 10 minutes. Then spoon the shea butter and melt for 10 minutes. Stir well until there is a smooth consistency and homogenous mass.

4. Cool the oils until the temperature reaches 90-95 degrees Fahrenheit.

5. Then pour the lye mixture into the pot with the oils. Mix well until there is a smooth consistency and homogenous mass.

6. Add the rose essential oil and pink soap colorant and mix well.

7. Pour the mixture into the molds. In 5 days take the soap out of the molds and set aside for around two or three weeks. Remember to wait until the process of the saponification will complete and then use the soap.

During the soap preparation process always use rubber gloves, goggles, long sleeves and breathing mask.

Cinnamon and Pineapple Soap

Prep Time: 80-85 minutes

Ingredients:

- 4 tablespoons pineapple scented oil
- 16 oz olive oil
- 16 oz palm oil
- 16 oz castor oil
- 25 drops cinnamon essential oil
- 1 teaspoon cinnamon
- 6 oz soap base

How to Make Homemade Soap:

1. Cut the soap base into small pieces and melt it in the microwave or in a water bath.
2. Then set the pot with the soap base aside and let it cool in the well-ventilated room for around 30 minutes.
3. In the pot, combine the olive oil, palm oil and castor oil and blend using a stick blender or in a food processor until there is a homogenous mass.
4. When the soap base is completely melted, add the oils mix and mix well.
5. Then spoon the pineapple scented oil and cinnamon essential oil. Add in the cinnamon and mix well until there is a smooth consistency and homogenous mass.
6. Pour the mixture into the molds. Let the soap batter cool for about 40 minutes. Place the soap batter into the well-ventilated room or on the balcony.
7. Gently remove the soap from the molds and cut it into bars. Set aside for few hours and you can use the soap. This soap will gently cleanse your skin.

Handmade Mango and Coconut Soap

Prep Time: 70 minutes

Ingredients:

- 4 oz mango butter
- 2 tablespoons mango fragrance oil
- 3 tablespoons shredded coconut
- 10 oz coconut oil
- 10 oz palm oil
- 8 oz castor oil
- 7 oz soap base

How to Make Homemade Soap:

1. Cut the soap base into small pieces.
2. Melt the soap base over the low heat for 10 minutes or place it into the microwave. Melt the soap base for about 15 minutes.
3. Meanwhile, in the pot, combine the coconut oil, palm oil and castor oil. Spoon the mango butter and melt on a burner for 10 minutes.
4. Then set the oils aside to cool and blend using a stick blender until there is a creamy consistency.
5. When the soap base is completely melted, add the oils and shredded coconut. Then pour the mango fragrance oil.
6. Stir until there is a smooth consistency and homogenous mass.
7. Pour the mixture into the molds. Let the soap batter cool for about 40 minutes. Place the soap batter into the well-ventilated room.
8. Slowly remove the soap from the molds and use it.

Orange and Honey Soap

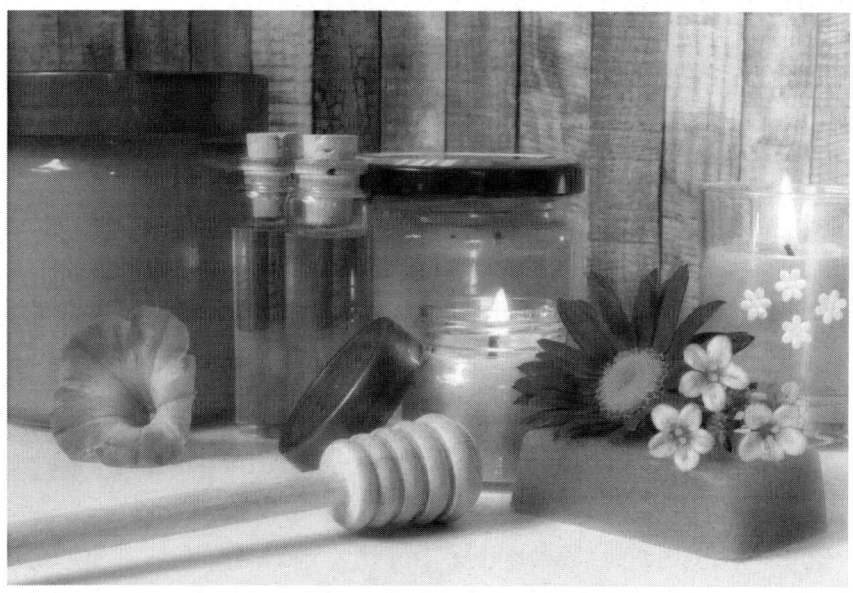

Prep Time: approximately 100-120 minutes

Ingredients:

- 20 drops orange essential oil
- 1 tablespoon orange zest, minced
- 4 tablespoons liquid honey
- 15 oz coconut oil
- 12 oz olive oil
- 11 oz palm oil
- 6 oz castor oil
- 9 oz distilled water
- 8 oz shea butter
- 7 oz 100% pure lye

How to Make Homemade Soap:

1. Slowly pour the pure lye into the water and mix carefully until smooth consistency. Keep stirring all the time or add some icy cold water, since it should remain cold. Don't forget to wear the rubber gloves, goggles and breathing mask, because the fumes will be produced during this process.

2. Set the pot with the lye aside and let the lye and water mixture cool for around half an hour. Place the mixture into the well-ventilated room or on the balcony.

3. In the pot, combine the coconut oil, olive oil, palm oil and castor oil and melt the oils on a burner for 10 minutes. Keep stirring the oils while heating.

4. Spoon the shea butter into the hot oils and melt it over the low heat for around 20 minutes until the butter dissolves.

5. When the lye and oils have similar temperature, slowly spoon the lye mixture into the oils. Use a stick blender to blend the mixture for 10 minutes until there is a smooth consistency and homogenous mass.

6. Then stir in the orange essential oil, liquid honey and orange zest and mix well.

7. Pour the mixture into the acrylic molds. The soap should harden, so keep it in molds for at least 24 hours before you can take your soap out of the molds and cut into square bars. Then place the soap in the well-ventilated room or on the balcony for few weeks.

Remember! During the soap preparation process always use rubber gloves, goggles, long sleeves and breathing masks.

Mild Coconut Soap

Prep Time: 70-80 minutes

Ingredients:

- 4 tablespoons coconut scented oil
- 14 oz coconut oil
- 12 oz palm oil
- 10 oz castor oil
- 1 tablespoon coconut butter
- 7 oz soap base

How to Make Homemade Soap:

1. Chop the soap base.
2. Melt the soap base in the microwave or in a water bath for about 5 or 10 minutes until there is a creamy consistency.
3. Then set the bowl with the soap base aside and let it cool for around 20 minutes.
4. In the pot, combine the coconut oil, palm oil and castor oil and blend in a food processor until there is a smooth mass.
5. Then combine the oils with the coconut butter and melt them on a burner for few minutes.
6. When the soap base is completely melted, add in the oils and coconut butter. Mix in the coconut scented oil.
7. Blend using a stick blender until there is a smooth consistency and homogenous mass.
8. Pour the mixture into the molds. Let the soap batter cool for about 30-40 minutes. It is recommended to place the soap batter into the well-ventilated room.
9. Slowly remove the soap from the molds and cut it into small bars. This mild soap will gently cleanse your skin.

During the soap preparation process always use rubber gloves, goggles, long sleeves and breathing mask.

Peach and Almond Soap

Prep Time: 60-70 minutes

Ingredients:

- 5 tablespoons almond oil
- 8 oz peach extract
- 20 oz palm oil
- 12 oz coconut oil
- 10 oz castor oil
- 11 oz shea butter
- 12 oz lye
- 3.5 cups of distilled water

How to Make Homemade Soap:

1. Slowly spoon the lye into the distilled water and mix well until there is a smooth consistency and homogenous mass. Cool the mixture for around 40 minutes.

2. Melt the shea butter on a burner for 5-10 minutes and then pour the oils and mix well. Spoon the peach extract.

3. Blend the oils mixture and lye/water mixture using a stick blender until there is a smooth consistency and homogenous mass.

4. Pour the mixture into the round molds. After 4 days take the peach and almond soap out of the molds and set aside in the ventilated place for about 2 weeks. Wait until the process of the saponification will complete and then use the soap.

During the soap preparation process always use rubber gloves, goggles, long sleeves and breathing masks.

Handmade Orange and Patchouli Soap

Prep Time: about 40-45 minutes

Ingredients:

- 20 drops orange essential oil
- 20 drops dark patchouli essential oil
- 15 oz palm oil
- 12 oz coconut oil
- 10 oz olive oil
- 7 oz pure lye

How to Make Homemade Soap:

1. Slowly spoon the lye into the water and mix well. Cool the lye for about half an hour. The fumes will be produced during this process, so wear the rubber gloves, long sleeves, goggles and breathing mask.

2. In the pot, combine the palm oil, coconut oil and olive oil and melt the oils on a burner for around 20 minutes. Then cool the oils.

3. When the lye and oils have the same temperature (around 90-95 degrees Fahrenheit), slowly pour the lye into the oils and mix well until smooth consistency and homogenous mass.

4. Then mix in the orange essential oil and dark patchouli essential oil. Blend the oils and lye mixture.

5. Pour the mixture into the molds and set the soap aside. Keep it in molds for at least 24 hours. Then take the soap out of the molds and cut into bars. Leave the soap in the well-ventilated room or on the balcony for few weeks and only then use the soap.

During the soap preparation process always use rubber gloves, goggles, long sleeves and breathing mask.

Homemade Pineapple Soap

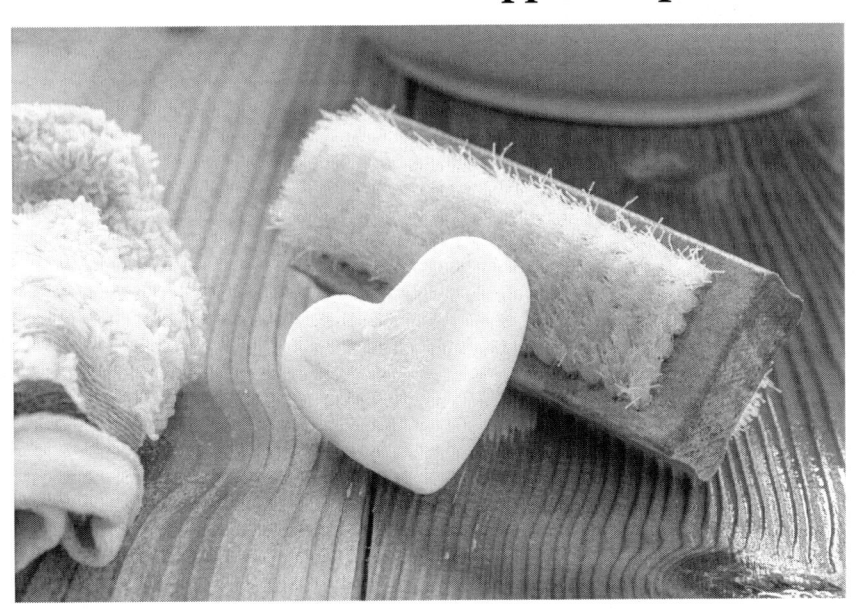

Prep Time: 40-55 minutes

Ingredients:

- 7 oz pineapple essential oil
- 2 tablespoons shredded coconut
- 5 oz cocoa butter
- 15 oz coconut oil
- 12 oz olive oil
- 8 oz palm oil
- 7 oz 100% pure lye
- 8 oz distilled water

How to Make Homemade Soap:

1. Slowly spoon the lye into the water and mix well until the lye dissolves. Remember that the fumes will be produced during this process, so don't forget to wear the long sleeves, rubber gloves, goggles and breathing mask.

2. Set the pot with the lye aside and let it cool until the temperature reaches about 90 degrees Fahrenheit. Leave the mixture in the well-ventilated place.

3. In a bowl, combine the coconut oil, olive oil and palm oil. Mix well and melt over the low heat for about 10 minutes. Add in the cocoa butter and melt over the low heat for around 10 minutes stirring all the time.
4. Combine the melted cocoa butter and oils with the pineapple essential oil and shredded coconut. Mix well until there is a smooth consistency and homogenous mass.
5. Then pour the lye and water mixture into the pot with the oils and cocoa butter. Blend all the ingredients using a stick blender until there is a smooth and pureed consistency.
6. Pour the mixture into the molds. After 4 days take the soap out of the molds and set aside for two weeks. Remember to wait until the process of the saponification will complete. After two weeks use the soap.

During the soap preparation process always use rubber gloves, goggles, long sleeves and breathing mask. This is important when you add the lye to water.

Pears-Almond Soap

Prep Time: about 40-50 minutes

Ingredients:

- 5 tablespoons almond oil
- 3 tablespoons pears extract
- 18 oz palm oil
- 14 oz coconut oil
- 11 oz castor oil
- 11 oz cocoa butter
- 7 oz 100% pure lye
- 7 oz distilled water

How to Make Homemade Soap:

1. Slowly spoon the lye into the water and mix well until there is a smooth consistency. The fumes will be produced during this process, so don't forget to wear the long sleeves, rubber gloves, goggles and breathing mask.
2. Then cool the lye and water in the well-ventilated place.
3. In a pot, melt the palm, coconut and castor oils for 10 minutes. Keep stirring to prevent the oils from burning. Spoon the cocoa butter and melt with the oils for 10 minutes. Cool the mixture.
4. Add in the almond oil and pears extract. Then pour the lye mixture into the oils and blend the oils and lye/water mixture using a stick blender until there is a homogenous consistency.
5. Pour the mixture into the square molds. After 4-5 days take the soap out of the molds and set aside for few weeks. Remember to wait until the process of the saponification will complete. After two weeks use the soap.

During the soap preparation process always use rubber gloves, goggles, long sleeves and breathing mask.

Handmade Goat's Milk and Coconut Soap

Prep Time: approximately 70 minutes

Ingredients:

- 1 cup of goat milk
- 12 oz coconut oil
- 11 oz olive oil
- 10 oz palm oil
- 10 drops coconut essential oil
- 6 oz lye

How to Make Homemade Soap:

1. Pour the goat's milk into the bowl or zip-lock bag and freeze for one day.

2. Cut the frozen goat's milk into pieces. Spoon the goat's milk pieces into the stainless steel bowl. Place the bowl with the frozen goat's milk in the sink filled with the cold water and ice cubes.

3. Slowly spoon the lye and stir well until there is a smooth consistency and homogenous mass. Remember that the goat's milk should be cold, so replace the water or add more ice cubes. Don't worry if the milk turns yellow. The milk should not turn brown.

4. Cool the milk in the well-ventilated room until the temperature reaches 90-95 degrees Fahrenheit.

5. In the pot, combine the coconut oil, olive oil and palm oil and melt the oils over the low heat for 10 minutes. Keep stirring the oils while heating to prevent them from burning.

6. Set the oils aside to let them cool.

7. When the milk and oils get cold, slowly pour the goat's milk and lye mixture into the oils.

8. Add in the coconut essential oil.

9. Blend the mixture using a stick blender for 10 minutes until there is a smooth consistency and homogenous mass.

10. Pour the mixture into the acrylic molds. After the 20-24 hours you can take your goat's milk soap out of the molds and cut into pieces.

11. Wait for about two or three weeks to enable the evaporation of unnecessary liquids.

During the soap preparation process always use rubber gloves, goggles, long sleeves and breathing mask.

Banana and Honey Soap

Prep Time: approximately 90 minutes

Ingredients:

- 2 medium bananas, cut into rings
- 3 tablespoons liquid honey
- 14 oz coconut oil
- 12 oz olive oil
- 8 oz palm oil
- 1 tablespoon shea butter
- 1 cup of distilled water
- 1 cup of lye (7-8 oz)

How to Make Homemade Soap:

1. Puree the bananas using the potato masher or stick blender. Pour some water and mix well.

2. Slowly spoon the lye into the water and mix well until the lye dissolves.

3. Keep stirring all the time, because the water should remain cold. Cool the mixture until the temperature reaches 90-95 degrees Fahrenheit. The fumes will be produced during this process, so wear the rubber gloves, goggles and breathing mask.

4. Slowly pour the lye into the banana puree stirring steadily until there is a smooth and homogenous mass.

5. In the pot, combine the coconut, olive and palm oils and shea butter. Melt the oils and shea butter over the low heat for 15 minutes. Keep stirring the oils while heating to prevent from getting burning.

6. When the lye and oils have the same temperature, slowly spoon the lye mixture into the oils. Then blend the mixture using a stick blender for 10 minutes until there is a smooth consistency and homogenous mass.

7. Mix in the liquid honey and stir well.

8. Pour the mixture into the molds and set the soap aside. The soap should harden, so keep it in molds for at least 24 hours before you can take the soap out of the molds and cut into pieces. Leave the soap in the well-ventilated room or on the balcony for few weeks and then use the soap.

During the soap preparation process always use rubber gloves, goggles, long sleeves and breathing mask.

Rose-Coconut Soap

Prep Time: approximately 70 minutes

Ingredients:

- 8 oz coconut milk
- 5 drops pink soap colorant
- 1 cup of coconut oil
- 15 oz olive oil
- 5 oz castor oil
- 7 oz palm oil
- 2 tablespoons rose petals
- 6 oz 100% pure lye

How to Make Homemade Soap:

1. Slowly spoon the lye into the coconut milk and stir well until there is a smooth consistency and homogenous mass. Remember that the coconut milk should stay cold. Set the pot with the lye and milk aside and let it cool until the temperature reaches 90-95 degrees Fahrenheit.
2. Meanwhile grind the rose petals.
3. In the pot, combine the oils and then melt them over the low heat for 20 minutes until there is a liquid and homogenous consistency. Keep stirring the oils while heating to prevent them from burning.
4. Set the oils aside to let them cool for around 30 minutes.
5. When the lye/milk mixture and oils are cold, slowly pour the lye mixture into the oils. Stir for 5 minutes and then use a stick blender and blend the mixture for 10 minutes until there is a smooth consistency and homogenous mass.
6. Then add in the rose petals and pink soap colorant and stir well.
7. Pour the mixture into the acrylic molds. After the 24 hours take the soap out of the molds and cut into pieces. Wait for about 4 to 5 weeks to enable the evaporation of unnecessary liquids.

Remember! During the soap preparation process always use rubber gloves, goggles, long sleeves and breathing masks.

Apple and Honey Soap

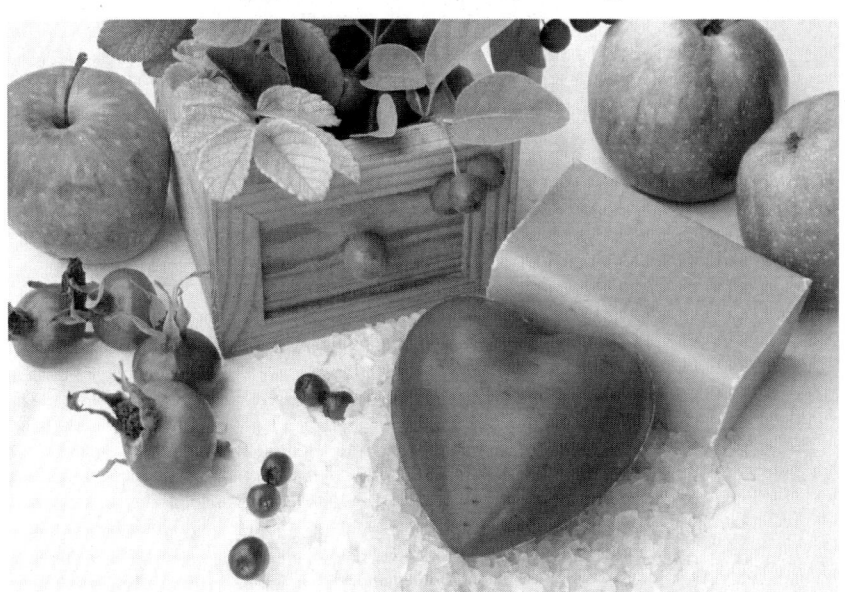

Prep Time: approximately 60 minutes

Ingredients:

- 2 apples, cut into rings
- 3 tablespoons liquid honey
- 12 oz coconut oil
- 11 oz olive oil
- 7 oz palm oil
- 1 tablespoon shea butter
- 8 oz distilled water
- 1 teaspoon citric acid
- 7 oz lye

How to Make Homemade Soap:

1. Puree the apples using the potato masher or stick blender. Pour some water and add the citric acid.

2. Slowly spoon the lye into the water and mix well until the lye dissolves.

3. Keep stirring all the time, because the water should remain cold. Cool the mixture until the temperature reaches 90-95 degrees

Fahrenheit. The fumes will be produced during this process, so wear the rubber gloves, goggles and breathing mask.

4. Slowly pour the lye into the apple puree stirring steadily until there is a smooth and homogenous consistency.

5. In the pot, combine the coconut, olive and palm oils and shea butter. Melt the oils and shea butter over the low heat for 20 minutes. Keep stirring the oils while heating to prevent from burning.

6. When the lye and oils have the same temperature, slowly spoon the lye mixture into the oils. Then blend the mixture using a stick blender for 10 minutes until there is a smooth consistency and homogenous mass.

7. Mix in the liquid honey and stir well.

8. Pour the mixture into the molds and set the soap aside. The soap should harden, so keep it in molds for at least 24 hours. Then take the soap out of the molds and cut it into pieces. Leave the soap in the well-ventilated room or on the balcony for few weeks and then use the soap.

During the soap preparation process always use rubber gloves, goggles, long sleeves and breathing mask.

Milk Soap

Prep Time: about 40-45 minutes

Ingredients:

- 3 tablespoons shredded coconut
- 10 oz olive oil
- 8 oz coconut oil
- 4 oz palm oil
- 7 oz cocoa butter
- 1 teaspoon sea salt
- 2 teaspoons Folded Coconut essential oil
- 1.5 cup of milk
- 6 oz 100% pure lye

How to Make Homemade Soap:

1. Freeze the milk in a freezer-safe container or zip-lock bags for about 6 hours.
2. Carefully spoon the lye into the frozen milk. Stir until the lye dissolves completely and then set aside.
3. Combine the cocoa butter with the oils and then melt on a burner for around 10 minutes. Keep stirring to prevent the oil and cocoa butter from burning.
4. Add in the sea salt. Stir using a stick blender until there is a smooth consistency and homogenous mass.
5. When the lye/milk mixture and oils are cool, pour the lye mixture into the oils and add the shredded coconut. Stir well.
6. Pour the soap batter into the soap molds. Then top with the sea salt. After the few days you can take the soap out of the molds. Place the soap in the well-ventilated room or on the balcony. Wait for about 4 to 5 weeks to enable the evaporation of unnecessary liquids until the process of the saponification will complete. After 5 weeks you are free to use the soap.

Remember! During the soap preparation process always wear rubber gloves, goggles, long sleeves and breathing mask.

Cherry and Coconut Soap

Prep Time: 40-50 minutes

Ingredients:

- 2 oz ripe cherries, pitted
- 4 drops red soap colorant
- 12 oz Cherry kernel oil
- 10 oz coconut oil
- 12 oz palm oil
- 7 oz olive oil
- 7 oz soap base

How to Make Homemade Soap:

1. In the pot, melt the coconut, olive and palm oils over the low heat for about 15 minutes. Cool the oils and mix them well.
2. In a bowl, mash the cherries using a potato masher. Then blend them using a stick blender until there is a smooth and "pudding-like" mass.
3. Meanwhile, dissolve the red soap colorant in some warm water.
4. Cut the soap base into small pieces.
5. Melt the soap base in the microwave.
6. When the soap base is completely melted, add in the oils mix, soap colorant, Cherry kernel oil and pureed cherries.
7. Mix well until there is a smooth consistency and homogenous mass.
8. Pour the mixture into the molds. Let the soap batter cool for about half an hour and then leave the soap batter.
9. After at least few hours carefully remove the soap from the molds and use the soap.

Activated Charcoal Soap

Prep Time: approximately 40-50 minutes

Ingredients:

- 2 tablespoons activated charcoal
- 13 oz olive oil
- 12 oz coconut oil
- 5 oz castor oil
- 7 oz cocoa butter
- 2 teaspoons sea salt
- 7 oz water
- 6 oz 100% pure lye

How to Make Homemade Soap:

1. Freeze the milk in a freezer-safe container for 8 hours.
2. Slowly spoon the lye into the frozen milk and stir slowly. Stir well until the lye dissolves completely and the set aside.
3. Combine the cocoa butter with the olive oil, coconut oil and castor oil. Then melt the oils over the low heat for around 20 minutes. Keep stirring to prevent the oil and cocoa butter from burning.
4. Blend using a stick blender until there is a smooth consistency and homogenous mass.
5. When the lye/milk mixture and oils are cool, add the lye mixture to the oils. Stir well.
6. Pour the soap into the bowl. Add the activated charcoal and blend well using a stick blender.
7. Pour the activated charcoal soap batter into the soap molds. Then top with the salt. After 2 days take the soap out of the molds. Leave the soap in the well-ventilated room or on the balcony. Wait for about 4 to 5 weeks to enable the evaporation of unnecessary liquids and until the process of the saponification will complete. Then you are free to use the soap.

Remember! During the soap preparation process always wear rubber gloves, goggles, long sleeves and breathing mask.

Gooseberry Soap

Prep Time: 40-45 minutes

Ingredients:

- 5 oz ripe and fresh gooseberries
- 5 drops green soap colorant
- 13 oz olive oil
- 10 oz palm oil
- 6 oz castor oil
- 7 oz soap base

How to Make Homemade Soap:

1. In the pot, combine the olive oil, palm oil and castor oil and melt the oils over the low heat for about 20 minutes. Blend the oils using a stick blender until there is a homogenous mass.

2. In a food processor, puree the gooseberries until there is a homogenous and "pudding-like" mass.

3. Dissolve the green soap colorant in some water.

4. Cut the soap base into small pieces.

5. Melt the soap base in the microwave or in a pot on a burner for about 15 minutes.

6. When the soap base is completely melted, add in the oils mix, soap colorant and pureed gooseberries.

7. Mix well until there is a smooth consistency and homogenous mass.

8. Pour the mixture into the molds. Let the soap batter cool for about half an hour. Place the soap batter into the well-ventilated room or on the balcony.

9. After 4 hours take the soap out of the molds and cut it into bars. Now you are free to use the gooseberry soap.

Remember! During the soap preparation process always use rubber gloves, goggles, long sleeves and breathing mask.

Mild Carrot Soap

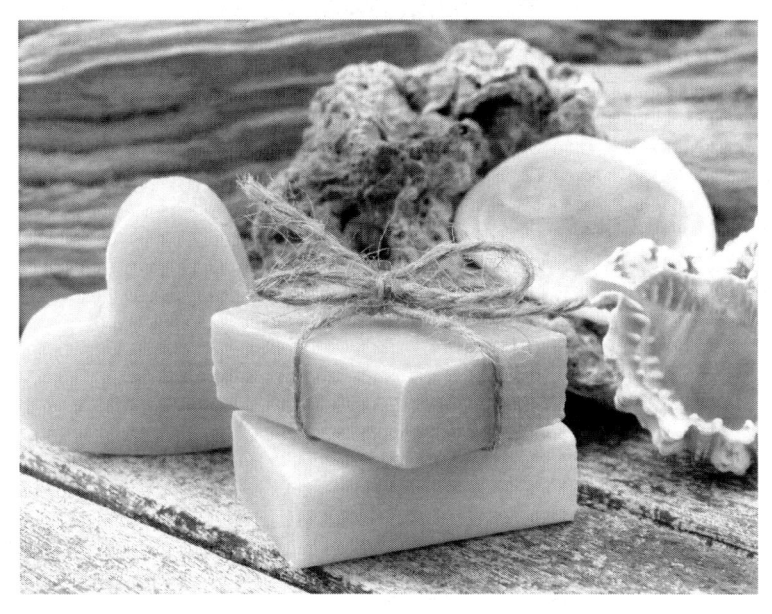

Prep Time: approximately 60 minutes

Ingredients:

- 10 oz cocoa butter
- 4 medium carrots, peeled and diced
- 14 oz coconut oil
- 12 oz olive oil
- 10 oz castor oil
- 8 oz distilled water
- 8 oz 100% pure lye

How to Make Homemade Soap:

1. In a pot, cook the carrots over the medium heat for around 20 minutes. Then mash the carrots with some cooking water using a potato masher or blend using a stick blender until there is a homogenous mass. Spoon the carrots into the stainless steel bowl and set aside to cool.

2. Place the stainless steel bowl with the carrots puree into the sink filled with the cold water and ice cubes. Slowly pour the lye into the carrots puree and water mix and stir well until the lye dissolves completely. Set the lye and carrots puree mixture aside to let it cool. Place the lye into the well-ventilated room or on the balcony. The main idea is to let it cool until the temperature will be lower than 95 degrees Fahrenheit.

3. Combine the cocoa butter with the coconut, olive and castor oils. Melt them over the low heat for around 20 minutes. Keep stirring to prevent the oils from burning.

4. When the lye/carrots puree mixture and oils are cool, pour the lye /puree mixture into the oils. Stir for 10 minutes until there is a smooth consistency.

5. Blend using a stick blender until there is a smooth consistency and homogenous mass.

6. Pour the mixture into the soap molds. After the 24 hours you can take your soap out of the molds and cut into pieces. Place the soap into the well-ventilated room or on the balcony. Wait for about 4 to 5 weeks to enable the evaporation of unnecessary liquids and until the process of the saponification will complete and then you are free to use your soap.

During the soap preparation process always wear rubber gloves, goggles, long sleeves and breathing mask.

Handmade Coffee Soap

Prep Time: about 40-50 minutes

Ingredients:

- 5 oz coffee grounds
- 6 oz coconut oil
- 6 oz olive oil
- 5 oz soybean oil
- 4 oz palm oil
- 6 oz water
- 5 oz lye

How to Make Homemade Soap:

1. Slowly spoon the lye into the water mix and stir well until the lye dissolves. Them add in the coffee grounds and mix well.
2. Set the pot with the lye and coffee aside for half an hour until the lye temperature reaches 95 degrees Fahrenheit. Place the lye and coffee into the well-ventilated room.
3. In the pot, heat the coconut, olive, soybean and palm oils and then melt them for 20 minutes.
4. Pour the lye and coffee mixture into the oils. Stir for 10 minutes until there is a smooth consistency and homogenous mass.
5. Pour the mixture into the soap molds. After the 24 hours take your soap out of the molds and cut into pieces. Leave the soap in the well-ventilated room or on the balcony. Wait for about 3 to 5 weeks to enable the evaporation of unnecessary liquids, until the process of the saponification will complete.

During the soap preparation process always wear rubber gloves, goggles, long sleeves and breathing mask.

Lemon Soap for Dry Skin

Prep Time: approximately 50-60 minutes

Ingredients:

- 3 tablespoons lemon zest, minced
- 5 oz lemon essential oil
- 15 oz olive oil
- 7 oz shea butter
- 10 oz grease
- 12 oz 100% pure lye – 5-7% superfat
- 1.5 cup of distilled water

How to Make Homemade Soap:

1. In a bowl, pour the water over the minced lemon zest. Use a spatula or spoon to stir well.

2. Slowly spoon the lye into the water and mix well until the lye dissolves completely. Remember that the fumes will be produced during this process, so don't forget to wear the rubber gloves, goggles and breathing mask.

3. Set the pot with the lye aside and let it cool. Leave the mixture into the well-ventilated place.

4. Meanwhile, in a pot, combine the olive oil, shea butter and grease and melt the soap ingredients on a burner for around 15 minutes stirring all the time.

5. Add in the lemon essential oil and mix well until there is a smooth consistency.

6. Then pour the lye and water mixture into the pot with the oils. Blend all the ingredients using the stick blender until there is a smooth and pureed batter consistency.

7. Pour the mixture into the molds. In 4 days take your soap out of the molds and cut it into few square bars. Then set the soap aside for two or three weeks. Remember to wait until the process of the saponification will complete and then use your soap.

Remember! During the soap preparation process always use rubber gloves, goggles, long sleeves and breathing mask.

Grapefruit Soap for Clean Skin

Prep Time: about 40-45 minutes

Ingredients:

- 2 tablespoons grapefruit zest, minced
- 3 oz beeswax
- 7 oz palm oil
- 5 oz castor oil
- 5 oz olive oil
- 12 oz lard
- 2 tablespoons Peppermint essential oil
- 6 oz 100% pure lye
- 8 oz distilled water

How to Make Homemade Soap:

1. Slowly spoon the lye into the distilled water and mix well until there is a smooth consistency. Remember that the fumes will be produced during this process, so don't forget to wear the rubber gloves, goggles and breathing mask.

2. Set the lye and water mixture aside to cool. Place the heat resistant container or pot with the lye/water mixture into the sink filled with the cold water.

3. In the pot, melt the palm, castor and olive oils and lard over the low heat for around 20 minutes. Stir well while boiling. Cool the oils for about half and hour.

4. When the temperature of oils and lye/water mixture becomes the same (around 80-90 degrees Fahrenheit) carefully spoon the lye into the oils.

5. Blend the oils and lye/water mix using a stick blender until there is a smooth consistency and homogenous mass.

6. Spoon the grapefruit zest and pour the Peppermint essential oil. Then add the beeswax and stir well.

7. Pour the mixture into the molds. In 2 to 3 days you can take your soap out of the molds and cut into bars. Then set the soap aside for around 3 weeks. Remember to wait until the process of saponification will complete and only then use the soap.

Remember! During the soap preparation process always use rubber gloves, goggles, long sleeves and breathing mask.

Orange and Grapefruit Soap with Honey

Prep Time: 45 minutes

Ingredients:

- 2 teaspoons Orange essential oil
- 2 teaspoons Grapefruit essential oil
- 3 tablespoons liquid honey
- 2 teaspoons ground barley
- 10 oz cold beer
- 14 oz olive oil
- 11 oz coconut oil
- 7 oz castor oil
- 7.5 oz 100% pure lye

How to Make Homemade Soap:

1. Pour the beer into the container and keep in the refrigerator for few hours.
2. In a pot, melt the oils (olive, coconut and castor) on a burner for 15 minutes. Set the oils aside to cool until the temperature reaches around 80-85 degrees Fahrenheit, it can take up to half an hour.
3. Then pour the orange and grapefruit essential oils and mix well.
4. Next, slowly spoon the lye into the beer and mix well until the lye dissolves completely. The fumes will be produced during this process, so wear the rubber gloves, goggles and breathing mask.
5. Set the pot with the lye aside and let it cool for approximately 1 hour until it reaches 80-90 degrees Fahrenheit. Leave the soap batter in the well-ventilated place like balcony for few hours to cool.
6. Then pour the lye and beer mixture into the pot with the oils. Stir well.
7. Spoon the ground barley and liquid honey. Mix all the ingredients using a stick or immersion blender until there is a homogenous mass.
8. Pour the mixture into the molds. In 4 to 5 days you can take the soap out of the molds and cut it into pieces. Then set aside for two

or three weeks. Remember to wait until the process of the saponification will complete and then use the soap.

During the soap preparation process always use rubber gloves, goggles, long sleeves and breathing mask. This is important when you add the lye to water.

Apricot Soap with Lemon

Prep Time: 40-50 minutes

Ingredients:

- 2 tablespoons Apricot kernel oil
- 2 tablespoons Lemon essential oil
- 2 tablespoons liquid honey
- 7 oz distilled water
- 6 oz almond oil
- 13 oz olive oil
- 9 oz coconut oil
- 7 oz palm oil
- 7 oz 100% pure lye

How to Make Homemade Soap:

1. Carefully spoon the lye into the water and mix well until the lye dissolves completely. Remember that the fumes will be produced during this process, so don't forget to wear the rubber gloves, goggles and breathing mask.
2. Set the pot with the lye aside and let it cool until the temperature reaches 80-90 degrees Fahrenheit. Place the mixture into the well-ventilated room.
3. In a pot, combine the almond oil, olive oil, coconut oil and palm oil. Then melt the oils on a burner for 15 minutes. Set the oils aside to cool until the temperature reaches around 80-90 degrees Fahrenheit.
4. Then add the Apricot kernel oil and Lemon essential oil.
5. Pour the lye and water mixture into the pot with the oils. Mix well.
6. Spoon the liquid honey. Mix all the ingredients using stick blender until there is a smooth consistency and pureed mass.
7. Ladle the soap batter into the square soap molds. In 4 days take the soap out of the molds and cut it into pieces. Then set aside for two or three weeks. Remember to wait until the process of the saponification will complete and then use your soap.

During the soap preparation process always use rubber gloves, goggles, long sleeves and breathing mask.

Blueberry Soap

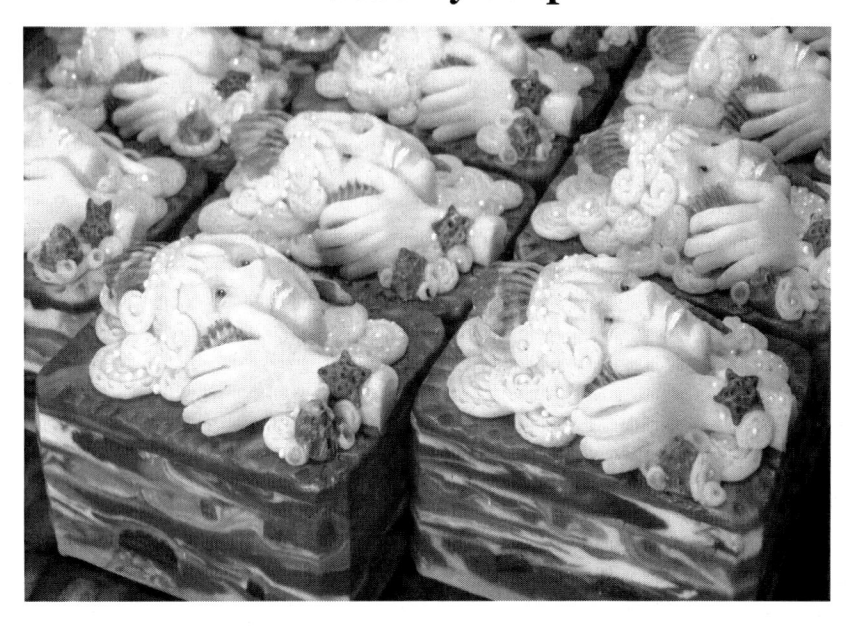

Prep Time: 40-45 minutes

Ingredients:

- 1 cup of blueberries
- 13 oz olive oil
- 11 oz palm oil
- 6 oz castor oil
- 7 oz soap base

How to Make Homemade Soap:

1. In the pot, combine the olive oil, palm oil and castor oil and melt the oils on a burner over the low heat for about 15 minutes. Cool the oils and mix them well.

2. In a bowl, mash the blueberries using a potato masher or fork. Then blend them using a stick blender until there is a smooth and "pudding-like" mass.

3. Cut the soap base into small pieces.

4. Melt the soap base in a pot over the low heat for about 20 minutes.

5. When the soap base is completely melted, add in the oils mix and pureed blueberries.

6. Mix well until there is a smooth consistency and homogenous mass.

7. Pour the mixture into the molds. Let the soap batter cool for about 40 minutes. Place the soap batter into the well-ventilated room.

8. Gently remove the soap from the molds and cut it into pieces. Now you are free to use the blueberry soap.

Yogurt and Avocado Soap

Prep Time: approximately 40-45 minutes

Ingredients:

- 2 cups of yogurt
- 2 avocados, pitted
- 15 oz coconut oil
- 14 oz olive oil
- 12 oz palm oil
- 6 oz 100% pure lye
- 1 cup of water

How to Make Homemade Soap:

1. Peel and then chop the avocados. Mash the avocados using the potato masher or fork.

2. Pour the yogurt into the bowl with the mashed avocados and blend the ingredients using the stick blender until there is a "pudding-like" consistency.

3. Pour the water into the pot. Then slowly spoon the lye into the water and stir well until there is a smooth consistency and homogenous mass.

4. The fumes will be produced during this process, so keep the water cold. Add a few ice cubes if needed. Keep stirring all the time, since the water must remain cold. Set the pot with the water and lye aside and let it cool until the temperature reaches 85-90 degrees Fahrenheit.

5. In the pot, combine the coconut oil, olive oil and palm oil and melt the oils over the low heat for about 15 minutes.

6. Set the oils aside to let them cool for around 30 minutes.

7. When the water/lye mixture and oils are cold, slowly pour the water and lye mixture into the oils. Stir for 5 minutes and then blend the mixture for 10 minutes until there is a smooth consistency and homogenous mass.

8. Then mix in the avocado and yogurt mixture. After you have mixed all the ingredients blend them well using a stick blender until you get a pureed consistency.

9. Pour the mixture into the molds. After the 24 hours you can take the soap out of the molds and cut into bars. Wait for about four weeks to enable the evaporation of unnecessary liquids and then use the avocado soap.

During the soap preparation process always use rubber gloves, goggles, long sleeves and breathing mask.

Raspberry Soap

Prep Time: 50-60 minutes

Ingredients:

- 0.5 cup of ripe raspberries
- 5 drops pink soap colorant
- 14 oz olive oil
- 11 oz palm oil
- 6 oz castor oil
- 7 oz soap base

How to Make Homemade Soap:

1. In the pot, combine the olive oil, palm oil and castor oil and melt the oils on a burner over the low heat for about 15 minutes. Cool the oils and mix them well.

2. In a bowl, mash the raspberries using a potato masher. Then blend them using a stick blender until there is a smooth and "pudding-like" mass.

3. Meanwhile, dissolve the pink soap colorant in some water.

4. Cut the soap base into small pieces.

5. Melt the soap base in a pot over the low heat for about 20 minutes.

6. When the soap base is completely melted, add in the oils mix, soap colorant and pureed raspberries.

7. Mix well until there is a smooth consistency and homogenous mass.

8. Pour the mixture into the molds. Let the soap batter cool for about 40 minutes. Place the soap batter into the well-ventilated room.

9. Gently remove the soap from the molds and cut it into pieces. Now you are free to use the raspberry soap.

Cheery and Grapefruit Soap

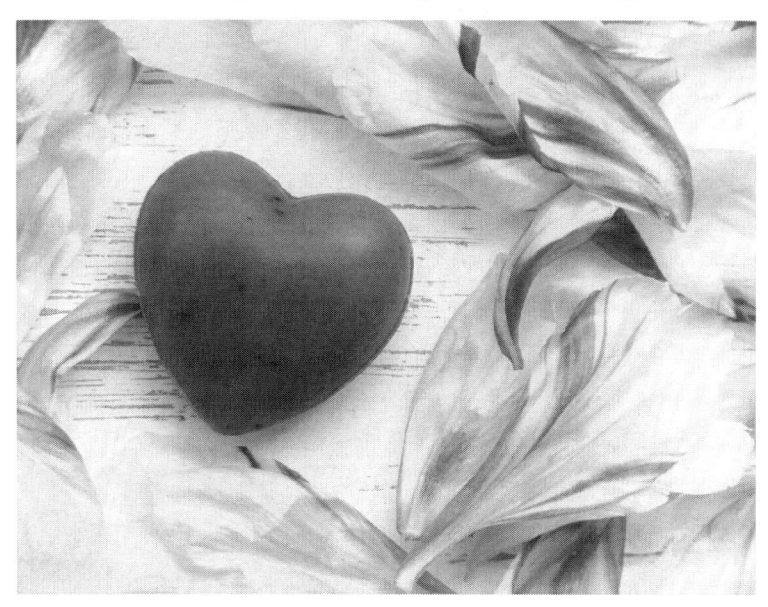

Prep Time: 40-50 minutes

Ingredients:

- 2 tablespoons Cherry kernel oil
- 2 tablespoons Grapefruit essential oil
- 1 tablespoon pink colorant
- 13 oz olive oil
- 11 oz coconut oil
- 7 oz palm oil
- 7 oz distilled water
- 6.7 oz 100% pure lye

How to Make Homemade Soap:

1. Slowly spoon the lye into the water and mix well until the lye dissolves completely. The fumes will be produced during this process, so wear the rubber gloves, goggles and breathing mask.

2. Set the pot with the lye aside and let it cool for few hours until the temperature reaches 80-90 degrees Fahrenheit. Leave the soap batter in the well-ventilated place.

3. In a pot, melt the olive, coconut and palm oils over the low heat for 15 minutes. Set the oils aside to cool until the temperature reaches around 80-85 degrees Fahrenheit.

4. Meanwhile, dissolve the pink soap colorant in some water.

5. Then pour the cherry kernel oil, pink colorant and grapefruit essential oil into the oils mixture and stir well.

6. Pour the lye and water mixture into the pot with the oils. Mix all the ingredients using a stick blender until there is a homogenous mass.

7. Ladle the mixture into the molds. In 4 to 5 days take the soap out of the molds and cut it into small bars. Then set aside for two or three weeks. Remember to wait until the process of the saponification will complete and then use the soap.

During the soap preparation process always use rubber gloves, goggles, long sleeves and breathing mask.

Conclusion

Thank you for buying this soap book. I hope this book was able to help you to prepare fragrant and beautiful homemade soaps.

If you are new in this field, this book will help you to start your soap journey. The recipes in this book are simple, and the process of preparing homemade soaps is explained in the simple way. We also added some more complex recipes. Those you can use, when you level of experience will grow and you will feel more confident. But never give up, always be open to learn and try new soap recipes.

Thank you again and I hope you have enjoyed this soap cooking book.

Manufactured by Amazon.ca
Acheson, AB